VITAMIN – D

DECODED

CONTENTS

INTRODUCTION

Vitamin D is a vital nutrient that plays a crucial role in maintaining overall health and well-being. Often referred to as the "sunshine vitamin," it is unique because our bodies can produce it when exposed to sunlight. This essential fat-soluble vitamin is necessary for a wide range of bodily functions, including bone health, immune system support, and maintaining proper cell growth.

There are two primary forms of vitamin D: vitamin D2 (ergocalciferol) and vitamin D3 (cholecalciferol). Vitamin D2 is mainly found in some plant-based sources, while vitamin D3 is the form produced in the skin in response to sunlight and is also found in certain animal-based foods.

One of the most well-known roles of vitamin D is its association with calcium and bone health. It aids in the absorption of calcium from the intestines and helps to regulate calcium levels in the blood. Adequate vitamin D levels are essential for maintaining strong and healthy bones, preventing conditions like osteoporosis and rickets.

Moreover, vitamin D has been linked to various other health benefits. It plays a critical role in supporting the immune system, helping the body defend against infections and diseases. Research has also suggested a possible connection between vitamin D deficiency and certain chronic conditions such as cardiovascular disease, diabetes, and certain cancers.

While sunlight is a natural and primary source of vitamin D, certain dietary sources can also provide this essential nutrient. Fatty fish (e.g., salmon, mackerel, and tuna), egg yolks, fortified dairy products, and some fortified foods are good dietary sources of vitamin D.

Despite its importance, vitamin D deficiency is prevalent worldwide, especially in regions with limited sunlight exposure or cultural practices that restrict sun exposure. People with darker skin are also at a higher risk of deficiency because melanin reduces the skin's ability to produce vitamin D in response to sunlight.

Health professionals often recommend vitamin D supplements for individuals with inadequate sun exposure, specific medical conditions, or those at risk of deficiency. However, it's essential to consult with a healthcare provider before starting any supplementation to determine the appropriate dosage.

Vitamin D is an essential nutrient that impacts various aspects of our health. Maintaining adequate levels of this vitamin is crucial for promoting bone health, supporting the immune system, and potentially reducing the risk of certain chronic diseases. Ensuring a balance of sun exposure, along with a diet that includes vitamin D-rich foods, can contribute to overall well-being and optimal health.

WHY VITAMIN D IS ESSENTIAL FOR YOUR BODY

Vitamin D is essential for your body due to its involvement in numerous crucial functions.

BONE HEALTH:

One of the primary roles of vitamin D is to promote the absorption of calcium and phosphorus from the intestines, which are critical minerals for building and maintaining strong bones. It helps regulate calcium levels in the blood and ensures that there is enough calcium available for bone formation and mineralization. Without sufficient vitamin D, the body cannot effectively use the calcium consumed through the diet, leading to weakened bones, increased risk of fractures, and conditions like osteoporosis and rickets.

IMMUNE SYSTEM SUPPORT:

Vitamin D plays a significant role in supporting the immune system. It helps activate immune cells and enhances their ability to fight off infections and diseases. A deficiency in vitamin D has been associated with an increased susceptibility to infections, and maintaining adequate levels of vitamin D may help reduce the risk of respiratory infections, flu, and other illnesses.

CELL GROWTH AND DIFFERENTIATION:

Vitamin D is involved in regulating cell growth and differentiation, which are essential processes for maintaining healthy tissues and preventing the development of cancer cells. It helps to control cell proliferation and prevent abnormal cell growth.

CARDIOVASCULAR HEALTH:

There is evidence suggesting that vitamin D may have a beneficial effect on the cardiovascular system. It may help regulate blood pressure, improve blood vessel function, and reduce inflammation, all of which contribute to heart health. Some studies have indicated that individuals with sufficient vitamin D levels have a lower risk of developing heart disease.

MOOD AND MENTAL HEALTH:

Emerging research has found associations between vitamin D levels and mood disorders such as depression and anxiety. While the exact mechanisms are not fully understood, it is believed that vitamin D may influence neurotransmitter function and brain health, potentially impacting mood and mental well-being.

MUSCLE FUNCTION:

Vitamin D is also involved in maintaining muscle health and function. It has been linked to muscle strength and coordination, and a deficiency may contribute to muscle weakness and an increased risk of falls in older adults.

ANTI-INFLAMMATORY PROPERTIES:

Vitamin D possesses anti-inflammatory properties that can help modulate the body's immune response. Adequate vitamin D levels may contribute to reducing chronic inflammation, which is associated with various diseases.

REGULATION OF GENE EXPRESSION:

Vitamin D can influence the expression of numerous genes involved in various physiological processes. It acts as a hormone that binds to specific receptors in cells, affecting gene transcription and influencing cellular functions.

It is worth noting that while vitamin D is essential for various bodily functions, excessive supplementation can lead to toxicity and adverse effects. Therefore, it is crucial to maintain a balance and seek guidance from healthcare professionals to ensure you are getting the right amount of vitamin D based on your individual needs and circumstances. Overall, maintaining adequate vitamin D levels through appropriate sun exposure, diet, and supplementation when necessary can significantly contribute to your overall health and well-being.

VITAMIN D DEFICIENCIES

CAUSES OF VITAMIN D DEFICIENCY:

Inadequate Sun Exposure: Vitamin D is often called the "sunshine vitamin" because the body can produce it when the skin is exposed to sunlight. Limited time spent outdoors or covering the skin with clothing can lead to insufficient sun exposure and, consequently, lower vitamin D production.

DIETARY INSUFFICIENCY:

A diet lacking in vitamin D-rich foods can contribute to deficiency. While some foods contain vitamin D naturally (e.g., fatty fish, egg yolks), many people rely on fortified foods or supplements to meet their vitamin D needs.

DARK SKIN TONE:

People with darker skin have more melanin, which reduces the skin's ability to produce vitamin D in response to sunlight. As a result, individuals with darker skin tones may be at higher risk of vitamin D deficiency, especially in regions with limited sunlight.

LIMITED ABSORPTION:

Certain medical conditions that affect the digestive system, such as celiac disease, Crohn's disease, and other malabsorption disorders, can impair the absorption of vitamin D and other nutrients from food.

OBESITY:

Vitamin D is fat-soluble, and excess body fat can sequester vitamin D, making it less available for the body to use. As a result, obese individuals may have lower levels of circulating vitamin D.

AGE:

As people age, their skin becomes less efficient at producing vitamin D in response to sunlight, and dietary intake may decrease, increasing the risk of deficiency.

Health Consequences of Vitamin D Deficiency:

BONE HEALTH ISSUES:

Vitamin D is crucial for calcium absorption and maintaining bone density. Deficiency can lead to soft, weak, and brittle bones, increasing the risk of fractures and osteoporosis in adults and rickets (a bone development disorder) in children.

INCREASED RISK OF CHRONIC DISEASES:

Low vitamin D levels have been associated with an increased risk of various chronic conditions, including cardiovascular diseases, diabetes, certain cancers, and autoimmune disorders.

COMPROMISED IMMUNE FUNCTION:

Vitamin D plays a critical role in supporting the immune system's function. Deficiency may lead to a weakened immune response, making individuals more susceptible to infections and illnesses.

MUSCLE WEAKNESS:

Inadequate vitamin D levels can affect muscle health and contribute to muscle weakness and an increased risk of falls, particularly in older adults.

MOOD DISORDERS:

Emerging evidence suggests a link between vitamin D deficiency and mood disorders such as depression and anxiety.

It's important to note that symptoms of vitamin D deficiency can be subtle and often go unnoticed. Common signs include fatigue, muscle pain, bone pain, frequent infections, and mood changes. If you suspect a vitamin D deficiency, it's essential to consult a healthcare professional for proper evaluation and to determine the most appropriate course of action, which may include dietary changes, sun exposure, or supplementation.

VITAMIN D IS REQUIRED FOR COMMUNICATION WITHIN YOUR BODY

Yes, vitamin D is indeed required for communication within the body. It plays a crucial role as a hormone that interacts with specific receptors in various cells, affecting gene expression and influencing cellular functions. This hormonal action allows vitamin D to regulate multiple physiological processes, contributing to overall health and well-being.

The primary form of vitamin D that acts as a hormone is calcitriol, which is the active metabolite of vitamin D. It is produced in the kidneys from vitamin D that is obtained from either sunlight or dietary sources. Once produced, calcitriol binds to vitamin D receptors (VDRs) found in the nucleus of cells throughout the body. This binding activates these receptors, leading to changes in gene expression and, ultimately, affecting cell behavior and function.

Some of the important functions of vitamin D in intercellular communication include:

BONE HEALTH:

As mentioned earlier, vitamin D plays a pivotal role in regulating calcium and phosphorus levels, which are vital for bone mineralization. By influencing the expression of genes related to calcium absorption and bone formation, vitamin D helps maintain bone density and strength.

IMMUNE SYSTEM REGULATION:

Vitamin D is involved in modulating the immune response. It can stimulate the production of antimicrobial peptides, regulate immune cell activity, and influence the inflammatory response. These actions contribute to the body's ability to defend against infections and maintain immune system balance.

CELL GROWTH AND DIFFERENTIATION:

Vitamin D influences cell growth and differentiation processes, which are essential for the development and maintenance of healthy tissues. By regulating genes involved in cell proliferation and differentiation, vitamin D helps ensure that cells function correctly and that abnormal cell growth is controlled.

CARDIOVASCULAR HEALTH:

Vitamin D may impact cardiovascular health by influencing blood pressure regulation, vascular function, and inflammation. Through these mechanisms, it may contribute to maintaining a healthy cardiovascular system.

NEUROLOGICAL HEALTH:

Emerging research suggests that vitamin D may play a role in supporting brain health and cognitive function. It may influence neurotransmitter function and neural protection.

ENDOCRINE FUNCTION:

Vitamin D can affect the function of various endocrine glands, including the pancreas, which produces insulin. This influence may be relevant to the regulation of blood sugar levels and diabetes prevention.

It is essential to maintain adequate vitamin D levels to support these intercellular communication processes and promote overall health. Vitamin D deficiency can disrupt these vital functions, leading to various health issues, as mentioned in the previous response. Regular sun exposure, consuming vitamin D-rich foods, and, if necessary, taking vitamin D supplements can help ensure that the body has sufficient vitamin D for proper communication and functioning. As always, it's best to consult with a healthcare professional to determine the appropriate vitamin D intake based on individual needs and health status.

WHAT CAUSES VITAMIN D DEFICIENCY

Vitamin D deficiency can result from various factors that either reduce the body's vitamin D production or impair its absorption and metabolism. Some of the common causes of vitamin D deficiency include:

Limited Sun Exposure: Vitamin D is often referred to as the "sunshine vitamin" because the body can produce it when the skin is exposed to sunlight. People who have limited sun exposure, either due to living in regions with little sunlight, spending most of their time indoors, or consistently covering their skin with clothing or sunscreen, are at higher risk of deficiency.

DARK SKIN TONE:

Individuals with darker skin have more melanin, which reduces the skin's ability to produce vitamin D in response to sunlight. This leads to a decreased efficiency of vitamin D synthesis and increases the risk of deficiency, particularly in regions with limited sunlight.

INADEQUATE DIETARY INTAKE:

Vitamin D can be obtained from dietary sources such as fatty fish (e.g., salmon, mackerel), egg yolks, fortified dairy products, and some fortified foods. People with poor diets or those who avoid these vitamin D-rich foods are at risk of deficiency.

IMPAIRED ABSORPTION:

Certain medical conditions that affect the digestive system can impair the absorption of vitamin D and other nutrients. These conditions include celiac disease, Crohn's disease, and other malabsorption disorders.

OBESITY:

Vitamin D is a fat-soluble vitamin, and excess body fat can sequester vitamin D, making it less available for the body to use. As a result, obese individuals may have lower levels of circulating vitamin-D.

AGE:

As people age, their skin becomes less efficient at producing vitamin D in response to sunlight. Older adults may also have reduced dietary intake, which increases the risk of deficiency.

KIDNEY AND LIVER DISORDERS:

Vitamin D requires activation in the liver and kidneys to become its active form, calcitriol. Conditions that impair liver or kidney function can reduce the body's ability to convert vitamin D to its active form, leading to deficiency.

MEDICATIONS:

Some medications, such as certain anticonvulsants, glucocorticoids, and weight-loss medications, can interfere with vitamin D metabolism or reduce its absorption, contributing to deficiency.

GEOGRAPHICAL LOCATION:

People living in northern latitudes, where sunlight is less intense and available for only a few months of the year, may be at a higher risk of vitamin D deficiency.

PREGNANCY AND BREASTFEEDING:

Pregnant and breastfeeding women have increased vitamin D needs, and if their intake is inadequate, they may become deficient.

Vitamin D deficiency can have significant health consequences, as discussed earlier, so it's essential to address the causes and ensure sufficient vitamin D intake through a combination of appropriate sun exposure, diet, and, if necessary, supplementation. Regular health check-ups and consultation with healthcare professionals can help identify and manage vitamin D deficiency effectively.

VITAMIN D DEFICIENCY SYMPTOMS

Vitamin D deficiency can lead to a wide range of symptoms, some of which may be subtle and easily overlooked. The severity of the symptoms can vary depending on the extent of the deficiency and the individual's overall health.

BONE PAIN AND MUSCLE WEAKNESS:

Vitamin D plays a vital role in calcium absorption and bone health. Deficiency can lead to a condition known as osteomalacia in adults, which causes weak and painful bones. Muscle weakness and an increased risk of falls may also occur due to the impact on muscle function.

JOINT PAIN:

Vitamin D deficiency can contribute to joint pain and discomfort.

FATIGUE AND WEAKNESS:

Feeling constantly tired and weak can be a sign of vitamin D deficiency.

MOOD CHANGES:

Some studies have suggested a link between vitamin D deficiency and mood disorders, such as depression and anxiety.

FREQUENT INFECTIONS:

Vitamin D is involved in supporting the immune system. Deficiency may result in an increased susceptibility to infections and illnesses.

DELAYED WOUND HEALING:

Poor wound healing or slow recovery from injuries may be a sign of vitamin D deficiency.

HAIR LOSS:

In some cases, hair loss may be associated with low vitamin D levels.

BONE DEFORMITIES IN CHILDREN:

In severe cases of vitamin D deficiency, children may develop rickets, a condition characterized by soft, weak bones that can lead to skeletal deformities.

IMPAIRED GROWTH IN CHILDREN:

Vitamin D deficiency can affect a child's growth and development.

It's important to note that these symptoms are not specific to vitamin D deficiency and can be caused by various other health conditions. If you experience any of these symptoms, it's essential to consult a healthcare professional for proper evaluation and diagnosis. They can perform a blood test to measure your vitamin D levels and determine if supplementation or other interventions are necessary.

Keep in mind that vitamin D deficiency can be prevented or treated by ensuring sufficient sun exposure (while taking care to avoid overexposure and sunburn), consuming foods rich in vitamin D, and, if needed, taking vitamin D supplements under the guidance of a healthcare provider. Regular health check-ups can help identify and address any nutritional deficiencies, promoting overall health and well-being.

THE POTENTIAL IMPACT OF VITAMIN D

DEFICIENCY

Vitamin D deficiency can have significant and far-reaching impacts on overall health and well-being. As an essential nutrient, vitamin D plays a crucial role in various physiological processes throughout the body. When there is insufficient vitamin D, several systems can be affected, leading to potential health consequences.

BONE HEALTH ISSUES:

Vitamin D is essential for calcium absorption and bone mineralization. Without enough vitamin D, the body struggles to maintain proper calcium levels, leading to weakened bones and an increased risk of bone-related conditions such as osteoporosis in adults and rickets in children. Osteoporosis can make bones fragile and prone to fractures, while rickets can lead to soft and improperly developed bones in growing children.

IMPAIRED IMMUNE FUNCTION:

Vitamin D is involved in modulating the immune system, and deficiency can lead to a weakened immune response. This may increase the risk of infections and make it more challenging for the body to fight off illnesses.

INCREASED RISK OF CHRONIC DISEASES:

Research has linked vitamin D deficiency to an increased risk of various chronic conditions, including cardiovascular diseases, diabetes, certain cancers (e.g., breast, prostate, colon), and autoimmune disorders.

While the exact mechanisms are not fully understood, it is believed that vitamin D plays a role in regulating processes related to these conditions.

MUSCLE WEAKNESS AND PAIN:

Vitamin D deficiency can lead to muscle weakness and pain, which can interfere with daily activities and contribute to an increased risk of falls, especially in older adults.

MOOD DISORDERS:

Emerging evidence suggests a link between vitamin D deficiency and mood disorders such as depression and anxiety. Low vitamin D levels may impact neurotransmitter function and brain health, potentially affecting mood and mental well-being.

IMPAIRED WOUND HEALING:

Vitamin D is involved in the wound healing process, and deficiency may lead to delayed or impaired wound healing.

DENTAL HEALTH ISSUES:

Vitamin D deficiency has been associated with an increased risk of dental problems, such as tooth decay and gum disease.

COMPLICATIONS DURING PREGNANCY:

Pregnant women with vitamin D deficiency may have an increased risk of complications, including gestational diabetes, preterm birth, and preeclampsia.

HYPOCALCEMIA:

Severe vitamin D deficiency can lead to low blood calcium levels (hypocalcemia), which can cause muscle cramps, tingling sensations, and abnormal heart rhythms.

It's essential to recognize and address vitamin D deficiency promptly. A simple blood test can measure vitamin D levels, and healthcare professionals can recommend appropriate interventions, such as increased sun exposure, dietary changes, or vitamin D supplementation, to correct deficiencies. However, supplementation should be done under medical supervision, as excessive vitamin D intake can lead to toxicity, which can also have adverse health effects. Overall, maintaining adequate vitamin D levels is crucial for promoting optimal health and preventing various health complications associated with deficiency.

FOODS THAT HAVE VITAMIN D

Vitamin D can be obtained from certain foods, and consuming a diet that includes vitamin D-rich sources can help maintain adequate levels of this essential nutrient. Here are some foods that are good sources of vitamin D:

FATTY FISH:

Fatty fish are among the best natural sources of vitamin D. Examples of fish high in vitamin D include salmon, mackerel, tuna, sardines, and trout.

COD LIVER OIL:

Cod liver oil is a potent source of vitamin D. It is available in supplement form and is also used as a traditional remedy for boosting vitamin D intake.

EGG YOLKS:

Egg yolks contain small amounts of vitamin D. Including eggs in your diet can contribute to vitamin D intake, but the amount is relatively low compared to other sources.

FORTIFIED DAIRY PRODUCTS:

Some dairy products, such as milk, yogurt, and certain cheeses, are often fortified with vitamin D. Check the product labels to ensure they are fortified.

FORTIFIED PLANT-BASED MILK:

Many plant-based milk alternatives, like soy milk, almond milk, and oat milk, are fortified with vitamin D to provide a dairy-free source of this nutrient.

FORTIFIED BREAKFAST CEREALS:

Some breakfast cereals are fortified with vitamin D to enhance their nutritional value.

BEEF LIVER:

Beef liver is a good source of vitamin D, but it is essential to consume it in moderation due to its high vitamin A content, which can be harmful in excessive amounts.

MUSHROOMS:

Some varieties of mushrooms, such as shiitake and maitake, naturally contain vitamin D. The content may vary based on how the mushrooms are grown and exposed to sunlight.

FORTIFIED ORANGE JUICE:

Some brands of orange juice are fortified with vitamin D to provide an additional source of this nutrient.

It's important to note that the amount of vitamin D in foods can vary based on factors like the animal's diet, the fish's species, or the production process. Additionally, while some foods naturally contain vitamin D, others are fortified with the nutrient to improve their nutritional profile.

For individuals who have limited sun exposure or are at risk of vitamin D deficiency, supplementation may be necessary. However, it's crucial to consult with a healthcare professional before starting any supplements to determine the appropriate dosage based on individual needs and health status.

HOW MUCH VITAMIN D YOU NEED

The recommended daily intake of vitamin D varies depending on age, sex, life stage, and certain health conditions. The guidelines for vitamin D intake are typically expressed in international units (IU) or micrograms (mcg). Here are the general recommendations for vitamin D intake:

Infants (0-12 months): The recommended daily intake is 400 IU (10 mcg) of vitamin D per day for infants.

Children and Adolescents (1-18 years): The recommended daily intake is 600 IU (15 mcg) of vitamin D per day for children and adolescents.

Adults (19-70 years): The recommended daily intake is 600 IU (15 mcg) of vitamin D per day for most adults.

Adults (71 years and older): The recommended daily intake is 800 IU (20 mcg) of vitamin D per day for older adults.

Pregnant and Breastfeeding Women: Pregnant and breastfeeding women have higher vitamin D needs. The recommended daily intake is 600 IU (15 mcg) for pregnant and breastfeeding women up to 70 years old and 800 IU (20 mcg) for those 71 years and older.

It's important to note that some health organizations recommend even higher vitamin D intakes for certain groups or in specific circumstances. For example, individuals with limited sun exposure, dark skin, obesity, malabsorption disorders, or certain chronic diseases may require higher vitamin D supplementation. Additionally, individuals who are at risk of deficiency should consult with a healthcare professional to determine their specific vitamin D needs.

Excessive vitamin D intake can lead to toxicity, so it's essential not to exceed the recommended upper limits, which are usually set at 4,000 IU (100 mcg) per day for most adults. However, the upper limits may be lower for infants, children, and pregnant or breastfeeding women.

To ensure adequate vitamin D levels, a combination of sun exposure, dietary sources, and, if necessary, supplementation should be considered. However, if you are considering taking vitamin D supplements, it is best to discuss your individual needs with a healthcare professional to determine the appropriate dosage for your specific health circumstances.

VITAMIN D DEFICIENCY DIAGNOSIS AND TREATMENT

Diagnosing vitamin D deficiency involves a combination of clinical assessment, medical history review, and blood tests to measure the levels of vitamin D in the bloodstream.

MEDICAL HISTORY AND PHYSICAL EXAMINATION:

Your healthcare provider will ask about your medical history, dietary habits, sun exposure, and any symptoms you may be experiencing. They will also conduct a physical examination to check for signs of vitamin D deficiency, such as bone or muscle pain.

BLOOD TEST:

The most common test used to diagnose vitamin D deficiency is a blood test to measure the level of 25-

hydroxyvitamin D [25(OH)D] in the blood. This is the primary form of vitamin D circulating in the bloodstream and reflects the overall vitamin D status.

INTERPRETING BLOOD TEST RESULTS:

Vitamin D levels are usually measured in nanograms per milliliter (ng/mL) or nanomoles per liter (nmol/L). Generally, the following ranges are used to interpret vitamin D levels:

Normal: 30-100 ng/mL (75-250 nmol/L)

Insufficient: 20-29 ng/mL (50-74 nmol/L)

Deficient: <20 ng/mL (<50 nmol/L)

TREATMENT OF VITAMIN D DEFICIENCY:

The treatment for vitamin D deficiency aims to restore adequate vitamin D levels in the body. The specific treatment approach may vary based on the severity of the deficiency, the individual's age, health status, and any underlying medical conditions.

SUN EXPOSURE:

For individuals with mild vitamin D deficiency, increasing sun exposure can help boost vitamin D levels naturally. Spending time outdoors in direct sunlight, particularly during the midday hours when the sun is strongest, can promote the production of vitamin D in the skin.

DIETARY CHANGES:

Including vitamin D-rich foods in the diet can help improve vitamin D intake. Foods such as fatty fish, fortified dairy products, fortified plant-based milk, and egg yolks are good sources of vitamin D.

SUPPLEMENTATION:

For individuals with moderate to severe vitamin D deficiency or those who cannot get enough vitamin D through sun exposure and diet alone, supplementation may be necessary. Vitamin D supplements are available in various forms, including vitamin D2 and vitamin D3. Vitamin D3 is considered more potent and is the preferred form for supplementation.

The dosage of vitamin D supplements will depend on the individual's age, the severity of the deficiency, and other health factors. A healthcare professional will determine the appropriate dosage based on blood test results and individual needs.

MONITORING:

After starting treatment, follow-up blood tests may be recommended to monitor vitamin D levels and ensure that they are within the target range.

ADDRESSING UNDERLYING CONDITIONS:

If vitamin D deficiency is due to an underlying medical condition (e.g., malabsorption disorders), treating the underlying condition may be necessary to improve vitamin D absorption and utilization.

It is essential to work with a healthcare professional to diagnose vitamin D deficiency accurately and develop an appropriate treatment plan. Self-diagnosis and self-treatment of vitamin D deficiency, especially with high-dose supplements, can be dangerous and may lead to vitamin D toxicity. A healthcare provider can guide you on the best course of action to optimize your vitamin D levels and overall health.

CONCLUSION

Sure thing! In conclusion, understanding the importance of vitamin D is crucial for overall health and well-being. This fat-soluble vitamin plays a pivotal role in various bodily functions, including bone health, immune system function, and cell growth.

Throughout this book, we've explored the sources of vitamin D, including sunlight exposure and dietary choices. Fatty fish, fortified dairy products, egg yolks, and mushrooms are among the foods that can contribute to your vitamin D intake.

It's essential to strike a balance, as both deficiency and excess can have adverse effects. Regular, moderate exposure to sunlight, a well-rounded diet, and, if necessary, supplementation under the guidance of a healthcare professional can help maintain optimal vitamin D levels.

Monitoring your vitamin D levels through blood tests and adjusting your approach based on individual needs is a proactive way to ensure you're meeting your requirements. Remember, each person's situation is unique, and consulting with a healthcare provider is the best way to tailor your vitamin D strategy to your specific circumstances.

By prioritizing vitamin D in your lifestyle, you're taking a proactive step towards supporting your bone health, immune system, and overall vitality. Keep shining, and may your health journey be filled with the sunshine vitamin's benefits!

Vitamin D is a crucial nutrient that plays a vital role in maintaining overall health and well-being. Often referred to as the "sunshine vitamin," it is unique because our bodies can produce it when exposed to sunlight. Vitamin D is involved in various essential processes, including promoting bone health, supporting the immune system, regulating cell growth and differentiation, and influencing gene expression.

However, vitamin D deficiency is a prevalent health concern worldwide, with various factors contributing to its development. Limited sun exposure, inadequate dietary intake, certain medical conditions, and impaired absorption can lead to insufficient vitamin D levels.

The consequences of vitamin D deficiency can be far-reaching, affecting bone health, increasing the risk of chronic diseases, compromising immune function, and impacting mood and mental well-being. It is also associated with muscle weakness, joint pain, and other health issues.

To prevent and treat vitamin D deficiency, it is essential to strike a balance between sun exposure, consuming vitamin D-rich foods, and, if necessary, considering supplementation under the guidance of healthcare professionals. Regular health check-ups and consultations with healthcare providers can help identify and address vitamin D deficiency promptly.

By ensuring sufficient vitamin D intake, individuals can enhance their overall health, reduce the risk of certain diseases, and support their body's optimal functioning. As vitamin D research continues to evolve, maintaining awareness of its importance and taking proactive measures to maintain adequate levels remains fundamental to promoting a healthy and thriving life.

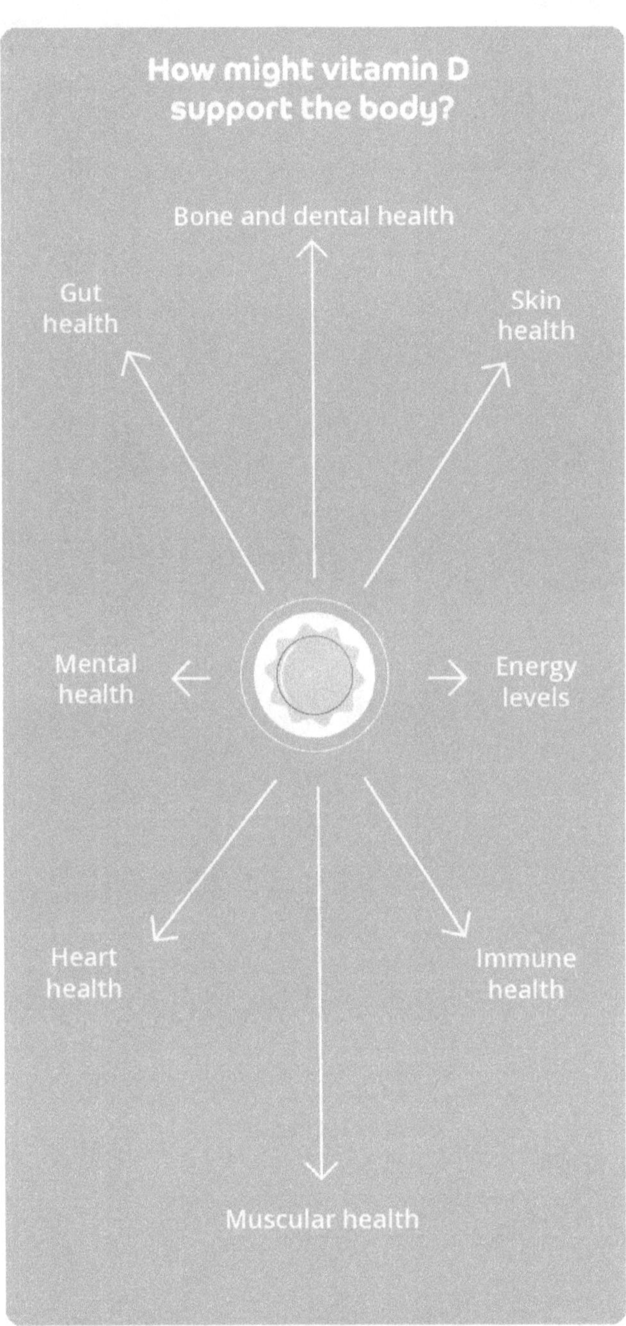

How might vitamin D support the body?
Bone and dental health
Gut health
Skin health
Mental health
Energy levels
Heart health
Immune health
Muscular health

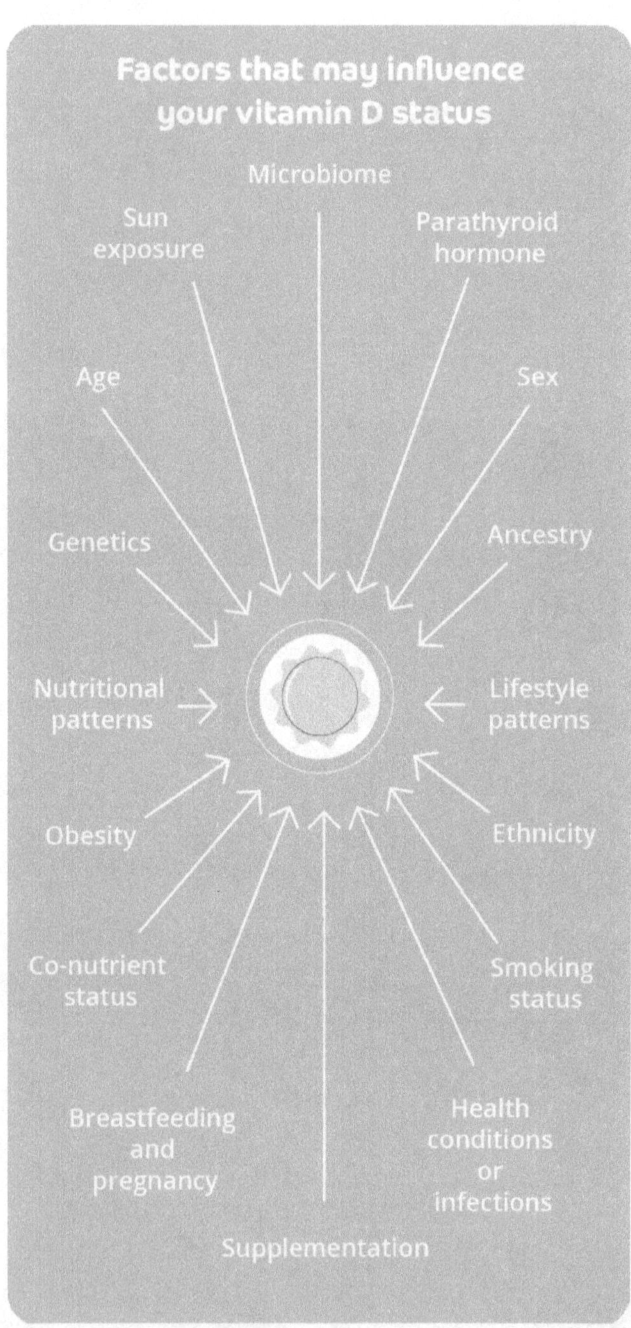

Factors that may influence your vitamin D status
Microbiome
Sun exposure
Parathyroid hormone
Age
Sex
Genetics
Ancestry
Nutritional patterns
Lifestyle patterns
Obesity
Ethnicity
Co-nutrient status
Smoking status
Breastfeeding and pregnancy
Health conditions or infections
Supplementation

Food item	1 Portion size	µg in portions	IU in portions
Cod liver oil	1 tsp	11.3 µg	452 IU
Farmed salmon	100g	7.8 µg	312 IU
Outdoor/ UV grown mushrooms	100g	3.25-11.2 µg	120-450 IU
Tinned tuna in oil	100g	6.7 µg	268 IU
Hard boiled egg	1 lrg	1.1 µg	44 IU
Lambs liver, fried	100g	0.9 µg	36 IU
Beef stewing steak	100g	0.6 µg	24 IU

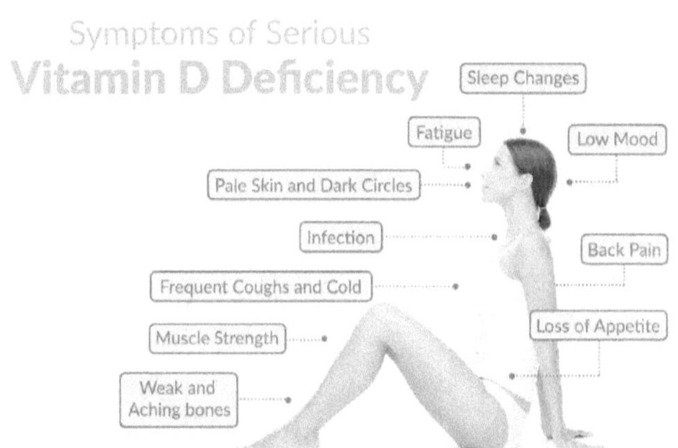

RECOMMENDED AMOUNTS OF
Vitamin D

AGE	MALE	FEMALE	PREGNANCY	LACTATION
0-12 months*	10 mcg (400 IU)	10 mcg (400 IU)		
1-13 years	15 mcg (600 IU)	15 mcg (600 IU)		
14-18 years	15 mcg (600 IU)	15 mcg (600 IU)	15 mcg (600 IU)	15 mcg (600 IU)
19-50 years	15 mcg (600 IU)	15 mcg (600 IU)	15 mcg (600 IU)	15 mcg (600 IU)
51-70 years	15 mcg (600 IU)	15 mcg (600 IU)		
>70 years	20 mcg (800 IU)	20 mcg (800 IU)		

*Adequate Intake (AI)

VITAMIN D DEFICIENCY
Affects Every Part of the Body

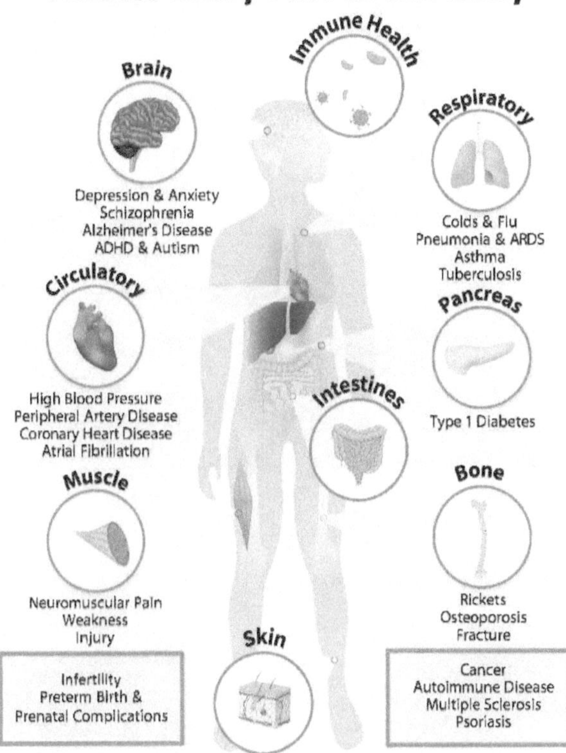